FIND

YOUR

WAY

Caring for yourself
while
caring for someone else

Verran Townsend

Published by Rippling Print

First published in Great Britain in 2019

© Verran Townsend 2019

The right of Verran Townsend to be identified as author of this work has been asserted by him in accordance with the Copyright Designs and Patents Act 1988.

ISBN 978-1-9161403-0-1

Dedicated to Karen
with deep love and gratitude.

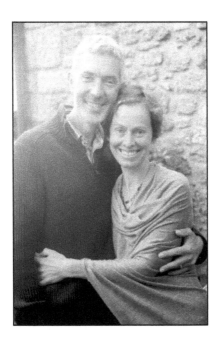

May this book help all who
care for others to live the
lives they share to the full,
embracing every moment.

Introduction

A year and a half after we met, we found a lump. Eight and a half years later my beautiful wife Karen died.

This book contains everything I found that helped me while caring for Karen, a positive ripple flowing from the immensely challenging, yet life enriching experience that we shared.

Whenever I discovered a new way to do something, or a new way of thinking, or being that worked for me, I wrote it down in a notebook. Page by page, that notebook became this book - a collection of reminders that helped me time and time again, and especially when I was struggling.

They still help me today, and I hope that they will help you too.

Try whatever catches your eye, whatever makes sense to you in your heart. Notice whenever you find a new way that works for you, and add to this book, or create your own, and keep it nearby.

May these thoughts help you to adapt, and to grow, and to find **your** way.

Your way to truly be with those that you care for, to nurture your own peace of mind, and to create the space you need for you.

With love,

Verran.

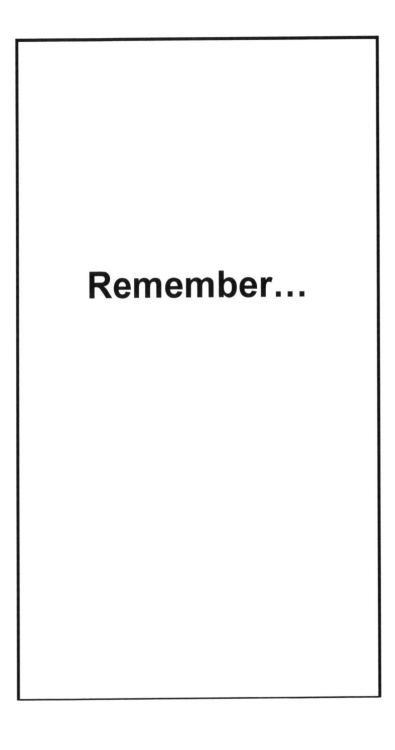

Remember...

You may not be able
to fix anything,
but you can
be with Karen,
alongside her,
all the way.

Start every day
by going outside
and before doing
anything else,
even if just for
a moment.

You can only do the
best you can do,
with love.

Let go of how you used to define yourself.

You're in a different place now, embrace it.

Once Karen has made
a decision about
her next treatment,
back her 100%.

If you're holding on
to thoughts of how you
would have chosen
differently, drop them.

Build, and keep on building a support network around you.

You'll need it.

What do you
need right now?

Ask for help.

What are you
grateful for?

Ask each other this
every day.

Speak from
your heart.

Always go with Karen
to see the doctors,
the nurses, and
the consultants.

A specialist's
opinion is only one
perspective.

Remind Karen
of this too.

Going to the hospital
with Karen will
impact you too.

Make sure your
support is also
in place.

Get involved – learn, research, share.

It feels good to contribute and help in this way.

Learn some
new skills that
can help with
Karen's healing.

Trying to be positive
all the time is tiring.

Give yourself a break.

It's ok
to not be ok
with what is.

Stop holding on
to the hope of a
positive outcome.

Dropping it will create
space to be with
what is right now.

Allow yourself to
dig in to the painful
thoughts and emotions
that come to you.

There's lots to
learn in there.

Saving for a rainy day?
Well here it is.

Allow the
money to flow.

Ask for a hug.

Let Karen help you
when you need support.

Take every opportunity to get to know your neighbours.

Join a men's group.

Meet up with
friends often.

Learn about mindfulness, you'll have many opportunities to practice it.

Spend as little time
in front of a screen
as possible.

Get enough rest,
especially sleep.

Have a little time to yourself each morning.

What food will nourish you right now?

Treat your body to the best quality fuel you can find, always.

Notice when you're struggling with unhelpful thoughts of the past or the future.

Take a breath, feel your feet on the ground, come back to the present, that's where you are.

Go to your
meditation class,
soak up the wisdom.

When you can't sleep, meditate on your breath.

If you still can't sleep,
send loving, healing
thoughts to Karen,
and breathe.

When it feels like there's too much going on, simplify.

What now, what next.

Just that.

Tidy up, and get rid of
stuff you don't need.

Are thoughts of what
could happen in the
future bothering you?

Notice when they come
and remember they
are just thoughts.

Nothing has changed in
this present moment.

It's quite normal to find yourself thinking about Karen's death.

Let the thoughts come and go, give them space.

What's the learning in them?

Remember that all
feelings come and go,
the most painful and
the most joyful,
and all in between.

Ever changing,
just like the weather.

You cannot know how others will react or behave towards Karen.

Their reaction is simply what is.

Be with that, just that.

Share your
thoughts
and
feelings
with others.

Keep in contact
with old friends.

Make time to
see your family.

Get specialist counselling just for you, lean on it often.

Find a place you
can go to when
you need to
scream.

Don't numb out.

Take responsibility for your own health.

The most important person for you to look after is you.

Only then can you really help Karen.

Don't spread yourself too thinly.

Get clear on what's most important and focus on that, and keep asking yourself what's most important now, and now, and now...

Keep asking for help,
even when you've
accepted more than
you feel you can
ever repay.

Accepting is a gift to
those who are offering.

It's tiring trying to work out how people could help you.

When someone offers, ask them how they would like to help.

Be gentle
with yourself.

Is what you're doing helping to improve your peace of mind?

If not, find another way.

What is weighing
heavily on you?

List everything
and sit with it.

Then find a way to
approach each one.

Free up space for all
that lifts you up.

What do you love to do?

Find time to do that too.

Collect wood,

Saw wood,

Stack wood,

Burn wood,

Watch the fire.

Go to your
yoga class.

What are you
naturally good at?

Do more of that.

Karen is stronger than you might think.

Let Karen know
how you're feeling.

Go on dates together.

Have fun taking
turns choosing what to
treat each other to
each time.

Surround yourself with
people, things, activities
that lift you up.

Avoid those that
drain you.

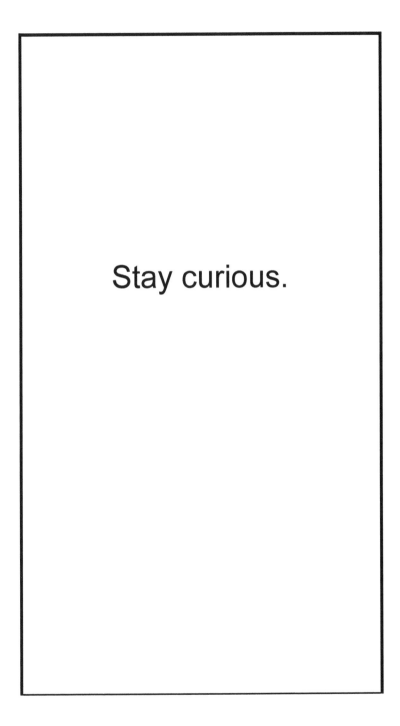

Stay curious.

Keep dreaming.

Have things to
look forward to.

Are you stuck in a rut?

Shake yourself free
and find a new way.

What advice would your
ancestors have for you?

Take a moment to tap
into their wisdom.

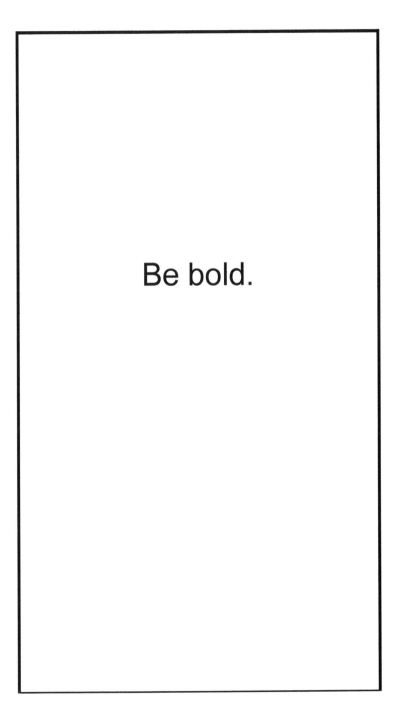

Be bold.

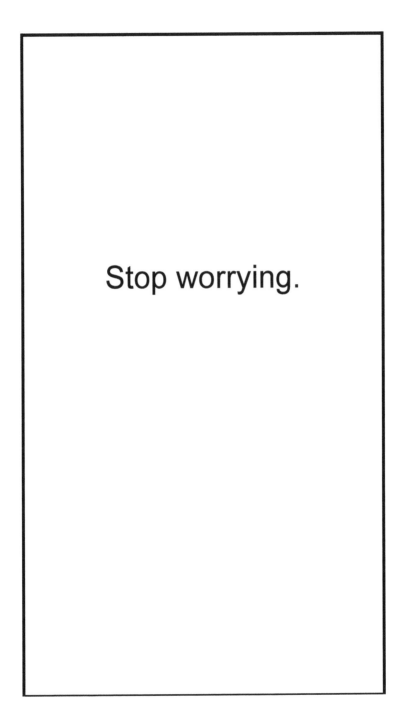

Stop worrying.

When you're frustrated with Karen and her illness, remember she's suffering too.

Allow your compassion for her to soften your frustration.

Keep on listening.

Have time away
from each other,
enjoy the space.

Enjoy being
back together again.

Caring is tiring.

Be careful not to
over-extend yourself.

Imagine yourself
years from now,
what advice would
your future self
have for you today?

Are you looking after
your own needs?

Keep on the look out
for tasty, and
easy to prepare meals.

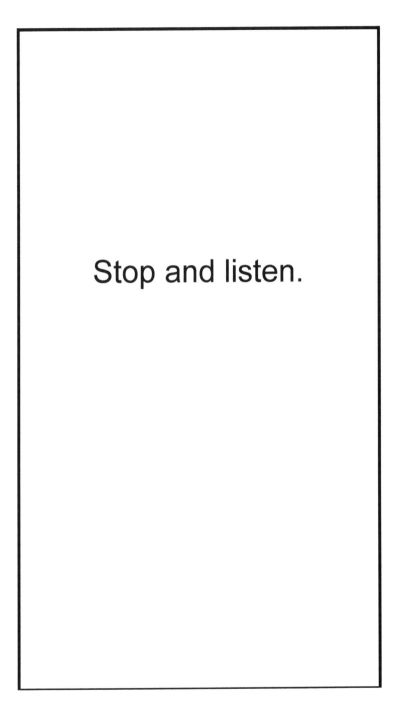

Stop and listen.

Watch the birds.

What message do
they have for you?

Spend time in wild
open spaces.

Lie back and
watch the clouds.

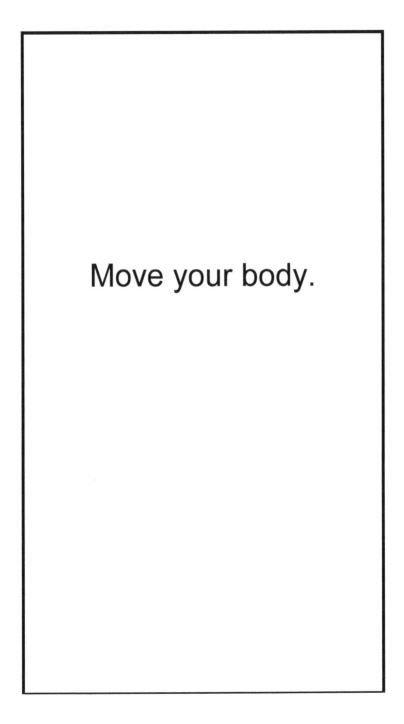

Move your body.

Go for a walk.

Don't use Karen's illness as an excuse for not following your path too.

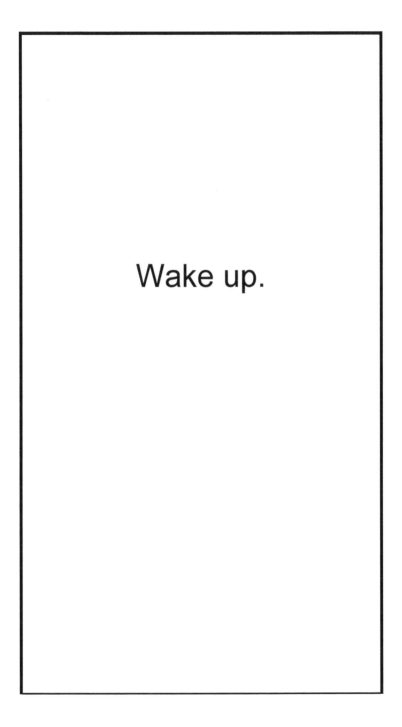

Wake up.

Stop eating or drinking
things that make you
feel crap.

Create space around you, get rid of anything you don't need or love.

Speak your truth.

You cannot know what others are thinking.

If you feel you need to know, ask them.

Celebrate when
something good
happens.

Reflect on the happy
times in your life,
especially
those with Karen.

Pause for a moment and see Karen for who she really is, cherish this time you have together.

This time is precious.

When someone really wants to know how you are, answer honestly.

They may have exactly what you need.

Reach out for help
when you're struggling,
even though it's the last
thing you feel like doing.

When cooking for two,
remember your body's
needs too.

Let go,
you're not
in control.

Talk about death.

Take notice every time it comes in to your life.

Allow any thoughts about how Karen might die to be present.

Feel the emotions, don't suppress them, let them be.

Your grief process has
already begun,
let it flow.

When strong emotions
rise up, let them,
be with them.

Cry.

If you've had enough of hearing about Karen's stuff, tell her, gently, and before the arguments start.

Don't cook when you're
tired and hungry,
have a snack first.

Making Karen a meal is a lovely thing to be able to do.

Let this thought help you when you've had enough of cooking.

Ask Karen what's most
important for her when
you're not sure,
and prioritise that.

Keep affection alive.

Don't distance yourself
to protect yourself.

Let go,

Let go,

Let go.

Keep doing the things
you love to do.

Go to your
pottery class.

Are you taking too much responsibility for Karen's wellbeing, and at your own cost?

Are you tired?

Take a nap, rest.

What can you do
differently today?

Look after your back.

When tense,
breathe deeply
into your belly.

Remember, most of the time Karen doesn't want you to fix anything.

She just wants to be heard, really heard.

Talk with Karen about her funeral, what are her wishes?

Find a place where Karen can feel safe to surrender, safe to let go.

There is nothing to fear
when death comes.

Being present at
someone's death
is a gift.

Help Karen to feel into where she is going next.

Leave nothing unsaid,
nothing undone.

Say goodbye.

Let Karen go.

Let her spirit fly.

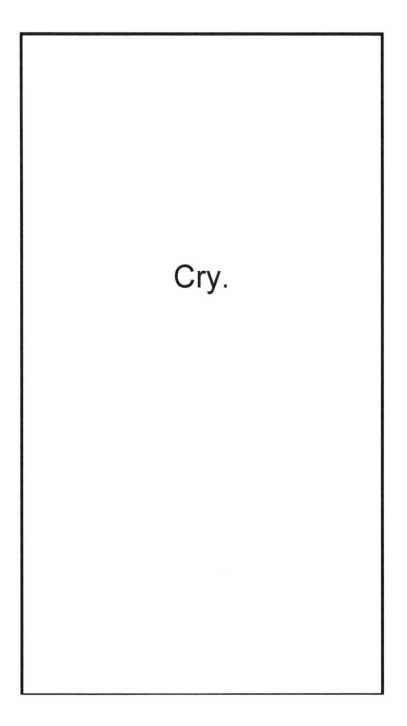

Cry.

Follow your heart.

Grateful thanks

Thank you Karen, my inspiration and partner in the creation of this book, absent in body but so very present in spirit. I love you.

Thank you to all our family, teachers, and friends who helped us both, in so many ways throughout our extraordinary journey together.

Thank you to all the healers, the doctors, nurses and care workers for your love and support.

And thank you to everyone that helped me in the creation of this book.

Lightning Source UK Ltd.
Milton Keynes UK
UKHW021423250819
348394UK00005B/42/P

9 781916 140301